Layman's Terms:

The Humorous Guide to Medical Misinterpretation

GREG WANNER, MS, PA-C

iUniverse, Inc.
New York   Bloomington

The views expressed in this work are solely those of the author and do not necessarily reflect the views of the publisher, and the publisher hereby disclaims any responsibility for them.

iUniverse books may be ordered through booksellers or by contacting:

iUniverse
1663 Liberty Drive
Bloomington, IN 47403
www.iuniverse.com
1-800-Authors (1-800-288-4677)

Because of the dynamic nature of the Internet, any Web addresses or links contained in this book may have changed since publication and may no longer be valid.

ISBN: 978-1-4401-7158-1 (pbk)
ISBN: 978-1-4401-7160-4 (ebk)

Printed in the United States of America

iUniverse rev. date: 9/8/2009

To my wife and family:

Thank you for everything. I could not have done this without your support and patience...especially the patience...you really had a lot of that.

Contents

Preface

We medical-folk speak a strange language. We use words like ipsilateral, hepatosplenomegaly, hysterosalpingo-oophorectomy, and esophagogastroduodenoscopy without even taking a breath. Somehow, we actually understand what these words mean. When speaking to a patient, however, our advice to "Schedule follow-up with the otorhinolaryngologist for further evaluation of your recurrent anterior epistaxis" usually results in a blank-faced, open-mouthed "Huh?" With so many bizarre medical terms flying around, it's no wonder that patients often misinterpret what we say…sometimes with humorous results!

The journey of *Layman's Terms* began nearly six years ago when I, as a physician assistant (PA) student and part-time emergency medical technician (EMT), started keeping notes of amusing medical misinterpretations. As the list quickly grew I realized how often medical words were misunderstood. The patient with self-diagnosed "ammonia in the lung" was entertaining but essentially harmless since it was easy to figure out that "ammonia" referred to "pneumonia." However, upon hearing a patient mistakenly refer to Lasix as "latex" when listing his allergies, I started to realize how problematic misinterpretation in medicine could be. I asked myself: "What if this patient were given Lasix by a healthcare provider who noted only the 'latex' allergy?" Thus, I decided to write this book both to amuse and to shine a humorous spotlight on the often funny, but potentially problematic phenomenon of medical misinterpretation.

To summarize, this book was written for the following reasons:

- Entertainment.
- To help healthcare providers recognize the types of medical terms that might be misunderstood, and to encourage providers to clarify these words for their patients.
- Entertainment.
- To assist the healthcare-student in understanding the misinterpreted medical language.
- Entertainment.
- A few other reasons that I can't remember right now...

While writing this book I researched the topic of misinterpreted medical terms, sometimes referred to as "medical malapropisms." In addition to conducting a survey (See "Research" chapter) I also scoured the entire world (i.e. several minutes of internet searching) to look for any information on the topic of medical misinterpretation. While I found a few websites and journal articles dedicated to this topic, I confirmed that *Layman's Terms* is by-far the most comprehensive book of medical misinterpretations and malapropisms to date... in the entire world...possibly universe. Ok, maybe a slight exaggeration...maybe.

I appreciate your decision to flip through *Layman's Terms*. For authenticity's sake I have painstakingly ensured that each included Term was personally witnessed by me or one of my trusted contributors. There's no need to make this stuff up! From "biscuit" to "vile duck" each Term was actually heard first-hand (or first-ear) straight from the misinterpreter's mouth.

In addition to being authentic, my goal was also to protect the privacy of the misinterpreters. Most of the material in this book has been drawn from my own healthcare experiences over the past eleven years. During this time I have worked, volunteered, and rotated through about fifteen different medical facilities along the East Coast. In addition to what I have personally witnessed, several colleagues have kindly provided Terms for this book. Their cumulative experience represents decades of healthcare exposure from across the United States and beyond. Thus, the material in *Layman's Terms* has come from tens of thousands of patient encounters and, in many cases, the Terms and quasi-quotes in this book have been heard from several different individuals. Therefore, nothing in this book should identify a specific person. Mr. HIPAA and I are friends and I'd like to keep it that way.

As a bit of a disclaimer, please understand that there is no disrespect or malice intended with this book. It is easy to see how many of these Terms and ideas could be misunderstood by patients, family members, and even healthcare workers. In fact, I recall mistakenly using several of the Terms myself. My goal with this book is to find some humor in the misinterpretation, not to ridicule the misinterpreter. (I'm sure my mechanic could develop a similar list with the various car-part names I have mispronounced or confused over the years. And yes, I *would* be ok with that.) Keeping my intentions in mind, if you are offended by any part of this book simply close the cover.

Still there? Good!

Now, let's get to the Terms! Please get comfortable, remove your stethoscope, take a deep "breff," and prepare to giggle…at least a little, I hope.

Greg Wanner

Acknowledgements

The following individuals have graciously donated medical Terms for this book. I would like to recognize and thank them for their contributions:

Al Castano, DO
Adam Coleman, MS, PA-C
D. Delcollo, PA-C
S. Dodd, PA-C
Mindy Elliason, MS, PA-C
Greg Gibson
K.S. Harres, MS, PA-C
Angela Kist, MS, PA-C
T. Love, MD
Jay A. Stiefel, DO, FACEP, FACP

Contributor & Reviewer:
Arayel Osborne, MD

Book-cover Artwork:
Julie Glaser Howery

Website host & Geek-consult:
Brian Wanner

I would like to extend a special thanks to Dr. Jay and Ms. Dodd for their constant vigilance during the search for Terms, to Julie for the perfect cover illustration, and to my wife, Dr. Arayel, for somehow finding the strength to deal with me during the compilation of this book.

Introduction

Welcome to *Layman's Terms: The Humorous Guide to Medical Misinterpretation*. The goal of this book is to humorously highlight how confusing medical terminology can be. Much like a foreign language, the language of medicine often requires translation from the medical jargon to a layperson's term. Patients and their family members frequently confuse or mispronounce a variety of medical words. Sometimes, the patient's version of the medical-speak is so incomprehensibly confused that a layperson-to-medical translator might be helpful to the healthcare provider. *Layman's Terms* is that translator...

This book is set up in a dictionary-like fashion to both enhance its readability and to give it the appearance of a credible reference...which, of course, it is not. The first few sections introduce the misunderstood Terms and use each in an example sentence. While each Term is "straight from the misinterpreter's mouth," many of the example sentences are dramatizations, based on a true sentence. To ensure that this book is fully, completely, totally, and undoubtedly HIPAA-compliant, some quoted statements have been changed to protect the misinterpreter.

As an overview, *Layman's Terms* is divided into several different sections:
- The Terms—Where each Term is introduced and translated.
- The Definitions—Selected Terms are further defined.

- One-Liners—A different type of misinterpretation, added for the sake of silliness.
- In Seriousness—An attempt at giving this book some sort of redeeming value.

Format:
In the first section, each Term is introduced in the following format:

Misinterpreted term   Actual medical term
[pronunciation]
"Example sentence using the <u>*Misinterpreted Term*</u> and *other Terms*."
See also: *other misinterpretations of actual term*

Because most of the Terms were spoken, rather than written, each Term is spelled phonetically. The pronunciation section is included to help clarify the misinterpreter's pronunciation, and add to the image of credibility. Just for fun (and to keep you pleasantly confused), some of the example sentences also include another Term found elsewhere in the book; these other Terms are listed in *italics*.

Styles of Humor:
I love dry, sarcastic humor. Although sarcasm is often negatively viewed as way to mock or ridicule, I feel sarcasm can take a more positive role. Sarcasm and irony are used in this book as tools to highlight misinterpretations and keep the reader's attention, not to ridicule the misinterpreter.

Unfortunately, identifying sarcastic statements from written text can sometimes be difficult and may lead to problems understanding an author's meaning. As an example, consider the following statement:

"When performing a throat exam, I love when the kid coughs in my eye…"

This could be interpreted in several ways:
(A) Literally—"I really do enjoy when children cough on me."
(B) Negatively—"I hate performing throat exams and hate children."
(C) Sarcastically—"While I dislike when children cough in my eye, I understand that it's part of the job… bring it on! (as I don my loogie-proof goggles)"

In case you missed it, this statement was intended to be interpreted as sarcasm. Because there is no specific literary indicator of sarcasm, I have used ellipses (…) in some cases to highlight a sarcastically-humorous statement, as in the previous example. I'm not sure if this is grammatically correct, but perfect grammar (or purfekt speling) was never my strong-point, so why start now?

As you read, please also keep in mind that I was a biology major in college. There's a certain stereotype I must live up to, namely, "Science folks can't do English." Thus, if you notice any grammatical errors or spelling mistakes in this book, they were surely put there on purpose, purely for effect. (That's my excuse and I'm sticking to it…)

Seriously:
And finally, a serious topic to consider as you read. Whether you're reading a confused Term, a bizarre statement, or my sarcastic commentary please do not doubt my deep underlying respect for the patient-medical provider relationship. This book is grounded in satirical humor. The sole goal is to entertain and inform, not to anger or offend. While this book is presented as a tongue-in-cheek guide to medical terminology, one must not lose sight of the true potential for clinical problems to arise from difficulties in communication. We, as healthcare providers, must continually strive to help our patients understand…even if we occasionally find humor in what they say.

Now we'll introduce the Terms. Enjoy!

Layman's Terms:

Anatomy & Physiology

The toof bone's connected to the limp note...

Biscuit   Meniscus
[bis-kit]
"When I twisted my knee, I tore my *biscuit*."

Brain storm   Brain stem
[breyn stawarm]
"I think he punched me in the *brain storm*."

Breeve   Breathe
[breev]
"With the asthma I can't *breeve*."

Breff   Breath
[bref]
"My chest hurts when I take a *breff*."

Chex   Chest
[cheks]
"I'm having *chex* pains and trouble *breevin*."

Circus   Cervix
[sur-kuhs]
"The gynecologist swabbed my *circus*."
See also: *service*

Circle spine   Cervical spine
[sur-kuhl spahne]
"The accident gave me whiplash of the *circle spine*."

Dick   Disk, vertebral
[dik]
"The MRI showed a herniated *dick*."
See also: *disco*

Disco   Disk, vertebral
[dis-koh]
"My back pain started when I slipped a *disco*."
See also: *dick*

Door   Dura
[dohr]
"They left the *door* open after my spinal tap and I got a headache."

Farnicks   Pharynx
[fahr-nix]
"I think I have another infection of my *farnicks*."

Fibia   Fibula
[fib-ee-uh]
"The fall broke my tibia and *fibia*."

Foreskin   Frenulum
[fohr-skin]
"The doc said Jimmy tore his *foreskin* when his mouth hit the stroller."

Gall duck   Gall duct
[gahl duhk]
"There's a stone stuck in my *gall duck*."

Gnomes   Nodes
[nohm]
"I got a sore throat and then some *gnomes* popped out of my neck."
See also: *limp note*

Gold bladder   Gallbladder
[gohld bla-der]
"This stomach pain must be from my *gold-bladder*."

Independix   Appendix
[in-di-pen-diks]
"I need surgery for a busted *independix*."

Larnicks   Larynx
[lahr-nix]
"The *larnicks* is near the *farnicks*."

Lemniscus   Meniscus
[lem-nis-kuhs]
"My knee is swollen from a torn *lemniscus*."

Lilac crest   Iliac crest
[lahy-lak krest]
"I've got a big purple bruise over my *lilac crest*."

Limp note   Lymph node
[limp noht]
"Before the fever I got these *limp notes* in my neck."
See also: *gnomes*

Lumbex   Lumbar spine
[lum-bex]
"I got a *disco* bulge at *lumbex* 4."

Mulder   Molar
[mohl-der]
"When I bit down, part of my *mulder* broke off!"

Postrate   Prostate gland
[poz-treyt]
"I get up five times a night cause of my floppy *postrate*."
See also: *prostrate*

Prostrate   Prostate gland
[pros-treyt]
"You need to do WHAT to check my *prostrate*!?"
See also: *postrate*

Retinal   Renal

[ret-n-uhl]

"The kidney wasn't working, so they put a stent in the *retinal vein*."

Rotary cup   Rotator cuff

[roh-tuh-ree kuhp]

"I twisted my shoulder and tore my *rotary cup*."

See also: *ruhtater cup*

Ruhtater cup   Rotator cuff

[ruh-tay-ter kuhp]

"I picked up a potato sack and tore my *ruhtater cup*."

See also: *rotary cup*

Scianatic nerve   Sciatic nerve

[sahy-an-at-ik nurv]

"I bent over and felt the pain down my *scianatic nerve*."

See also: *sonic nerve*

Service   Cervix

[sur-vis]

"My gynecologist made sure my *service* was ok."

See also: *circus*

Sonic nerve   Sciatic nerve
[sah-nik nurv]
"The pain shoots out my *sonic nerve*."
See also: *scianatic nerve*

Stumitch   Stomach
[stuh-mitch]
"My *stumitch* hurts, I think it's my *gold-bladder*."

Teef   Teeth
[teehf]
"Uh sure, I brush my *teef* everyday…"
See also: *toof*

Testamoid bone   Sesamoid bone
[tes-ti-moyd bohns]
"The doctor said those two things are my *testamoid bones*."

Theoraskic   Thoracic
[thee-or-ass-kik]
"I've had *theoraskic* back pain since I got beat up at the bar."
See also: *thoratick*

Thoratick   Thoracic spine
[thur-at-ik]
"I have a *dick* bulge in my *thoratick*."
See also: *theoraskic*

Tibula   Tibia
[tib-yuh-lah]
"The fall broke my *tibula* and fibula."

Toof   Tooth
[toohf]
"That *toof* hurts every time I eat Twinkies."
See also: *teef*

Tour-sell   Tarsal
[toor-sel]
"I started getting foot tingles after my *tour-sell tunnel* broke."

Turbine   Turbinate
[ter-bahyn]
"To help my sinuses the surgeon took out the lowest *turbine*."

Urinal   Urinary

[yoor-uh-nhl]

"I'm on antibiotics for a *urinal* infection.

Uterer   Ureter

[yoo-tuh-rur]

"The kidney stone is in my *uterer*."

Vile   Bile

[vahyl]

"The doctor said that my *gold-bladder* holds *vile*."

Vile duck   Bile duct

[vahyl duhk]

"Doc says I got a stone stuck in my *vile duck*."

Virginia   Vagina

[ver-jin-yuh]

"I think it's still in my *Virginia*…"

Layman's Terms:

Signs & Symptoms

History of the present illness? Good luck…

Abominable pain   Abdominal pain
[uh-bom-uh-nuh-buhl payn]
"I'm throwing up and have severe *abominable pain*."

Attention headache   Tension headache
[uh-ten-shun hed-ayk]
"Ahh, I need more morphine, my *attention headache* is really bad!"

Brewery   Bruit
[broo-uh-ree]
"I didn't find a carotid *brewery*."

Clog   Clot
[klawg]
"My period is so heavy I'm passing *clogs*!"

Diaree   Diarrhea
[dahy-uh-ree]
"My stools is just *diaree*."
See also: *diarear*

Diarear   Diarrhea
[dahy-uh-rear]
"It's all *diarear* from the bottom."
See also: *diaree*

Diluted   Dilated
[dahy-loo-ted]
"Check out my eyes, they're all *diluted*."

Enflaired   Inflamed
[en-flared]
"I think I have *enflaired* hemorrhoids."

Extended   Distended
[ik-sten-did]
"The doctor said my *stumitch* is *extended*."

Flatulations   Fasciculations
[flach-yoo-ley-shuns]
"I take medicine to help stop the muscle *flatulations*."

Gas reflux   Acid reflux

[gas re-fluks]

"When I eat too fast I get *gas reflux*."

See also: *reflex*

Inflation   Inflammation

[in-fley-shun]

"My shoulder *inflation* is getting worse but I can't afford to miss work."

Jaunince   Jaundice

[jaw-nanse]

"I have a history of yellow skin *jaunince*."

See also: *jarvis*

Jarvis   Jaundice

[jahr-vis]

"My grandson called me a pumpkin, I think I have *jarvis*."

See also: *jaunince*

Legend   Lesion

[lej-und]

"I got a *legend* on my penis."

Musagus   Mucus
[myoo-sah-gus]
"The cough is bringing up *musagus*."

Nawshet   Nauseous
[naw-shet]
"First I got *nawshet*, then I barfed all over."

Normer   Murmur
[nawr-muhr]
"I already seen a cardiologist for my heart *normer*."

Palpation   Palpitation
[pal-pey-shuns]
"Touch right here, can you feel my *palpations*?"
See also: *population, pulpitation*

Paste nosal drip   Post-nasal drip
[peyst nohz-uhl drip]
"I cough up thick white stuff from the *paste nosal drip*."

Population   Palpitation
[pop-yoo-ley-shun]
"I keep feeling *populations* in my *chex*."
See also: *palpation, pulpitation*

Pulpitation   Palpitation
[puhlp-uh-tehy-shun]
"Have you ever had chest *pulpitations*?"
See also: *palpation, population*

Reflex   Reflux
[ree-flecks]
"I can't drink coffee cause of my acid *reflex*."
See also: *gas reflux*

Retractions   Contractions
[ri-trak-shuns]
"I'm pregnant and I'm having *retractions*!"

Sored   Painful / sore
[sohrd]
"When I bent over my back got *sored*."

Sputem   Sputum
[spuht-em]
"I'm coughing up *sputem* and *musagus*."

Swold   Swollen
[swold]
"My legs is all *swold* 'cause I forgot my *water pill*."

Symbolic   Systolic
[sim-bol-ik]
"The pharmacy machine said my *symbolic* blood pressure was high."

Thyroids   Inguinal nodes
[thahy-roids]
"I got an STD, now my *thyroids* are all swollen."

Vagina   Angina
[vuh-jahy-nuh]
"No doc, I ain't got no *vagina*, just this chest pain."

Vomick   Vomit

[vah-mik]

"My baby has *vomicking* and *diarear*."

Welps   Hives / welts

[welpz]

"First he got a bee-sting, now he's got *welps*."

Layman's Terms:

Diagnoses

[Drum-roll] And the diagnosis is…

Absence   Abscess
[ab-suhns]
"My *absence* is *pussing*."
See also: *absets, ass cyst, pus bag, risen, spider bite*

Absets   Abscess
[ab-setz]
"The *absets* exploded and *pussed out* when I squeezed it.
See also: *absence, ass cyst, pus bag, risen, spider bite,*

Ace Pulari   H. pylori
[eys puhl-air-ee]
"The test found *Ace Pulari* in my stomach."

Amemea   Anemia
[uh-mee-mee-uh]
"The iron pills are for my *amemea*."

Ammonia   Pneumonia
[uh-mohn-yuh]
"I have *ammonia* in my lung."

Anemix   Anemic
[uh-nee-mix]
"I'm *anemix* from *low blood*."

Angerism   Aneurysm
[ang-ger-ism]
"My grandmother died of an exploded *angerism*."

Antrofee   Atrophy
[an-troh-fee]
"I stopped working out and my muscles *antrofeed*."

Ascysses   Cysts
[as-sis-ses]
"These ovary *ascysses* are giving me bad pains."

Ass cyst   Abscess
[ass sist]
"I got a huge *ass cyst* on my butt!"
See also: *absets, absence, pus bag, risen, spider bite*

Bopsee   Biopsy
[bop-see]
"They did a *bopsee* test for the skin *legend*."

Broncasma   Bronchial asthma
[bronk-as-muh]
"I can't *breeve*, I've got *broncasma*."

Cadillac   Cataract
[kad-il-ac]
"I couldn't see, so they took out the *cadillac*."

Ceaser   Seizure
[si-zur]
"Look, my arm is shaking. I'm having *ceasers*."

Cellyulitis   Cellulitis
[sel-ee-yuh-lie-tus]
"My skin's all *enflaired* from the *cellyulitis*."

<u>Chicken pops</u>   Chickenpox
[chik-uhn popz]
"My son keeps scratching at his *chicken pops*."

<u>Cirrhosis</u>   Psoriasis
[suh-roh-sis]
"Hey ma, show him the *cirrhosis* on your elbows!"

<u>Corporate tunnel</u>   Carpal tunnel
[kawr-per-it tuhn-el]
"My wrist hurts from typing, is it *corporate tunnel*?"
See also: *corporal tunnel, carper tunnel*

<u>Corporal tunnel</u>   Carpal tunnel
[kawr-per-uhl tuhn-el]
"I've got *corporal tunnel* in my wrist, sir."
See also: *corporate tunnel, carper tunnel*

<u>Carper tunnel</u>   Carpal tunnel
[kahrp-er tuhn-el]
"I think fishing gave me the *carper tunnel* pain."
See also: *corporate tunnel, corporal tunnel*

Diatickelitis   Diverticulitis
[dye-uh-tickle-itis]
"The stomach pain is from *diatickelitis*…hehe, ouch."
See also: *dieridiculous, dimeuhticulitis*

Dicker veins   DeQuervain's
tendonosis   tenosynovitis
[dik-er vehns ten-din-oh-sis]
"My wrist got *dicker veins tendonosis* from holding my baby."

Dieridiculous   Diverticulitis
[dye-ri-dik-yuh-luhs]
"This *dieridiculous* infection is ridiculous!"
See also: *diatickelitis, dimeuhticulitis*

Dimeuhticulitis   Diverticulitis
[dyme-uh-tic-yool-it-is]
"I don't eat nuts cause of my *dimeuhticulitis*."
See also: *diatickelitis, dieridiculous*

Diminished	Degenerative
<u>disk disease</u>	<u>disk disease</u>

[di-min-isht disk]

"The <u>*diminished disk disease*</u> gives me a little pain."

See also: *disintegrating disk disease*

Disintegrating	Degenerative
<u>disk disease</u>	<u>disk disease</u>

[dis-in-tuh-greyt-ing disk]

"My back pain is from <u>*disintegrating disk disease*</u>."

See also: *diminished disk disease*

Dramatic	Rheumatic
<u>heart disease</u>	<u>heart disease</u>

[druh-mat-ik hart di-zees]

"Ohh help me! I'm afraid I have <u>*dramatic heart disease*</u>!!!"

<u>Eczema</u>	<u>Emphysema</u>

[egg-zee-mah]

"I use the oxygen when my <u>*eczema*</u> gets bad."

Endomeseeosis   Endometriosis
[in-doh-mee-see-oh-sis]
"The <u>*endomeseeosis*</u> gives me a lot of *abominable pain*."
See also: *endrometosis*

Endrometosis   Endometriosis
[in-droh-mee-toh-sis]
"My <u>*endrometosis*</u> gets bad when I got my *flow*."
See also: *endomeseeosis*

Epsilepsie   Epilepsy
[ep-sill-ep-see]
"My mom has <u>*epsilepsie*</u>, ya know, *cesars*"

Eptopic   Ectopic
[ep-top-ik]
"They took out my tube from an <u>*eptopic pregnancy*</u>."

Esellititis   Encephalitis
[uh-sel-li-tayh-tis]
"My grandma had <u>*eselititis*</u> of the brains."

Exania   Anxiety
[ex-ayn-ee-uh]
"I'm afraid to go outside, my *exania* is so bad."

Exercise reduced   Exercise induced
asthma   asthma
[ek-ser-size ri-doost]
"He can't do gym because of the *exercise reduced asthma*."

Exotica   Sciatica
[ig-zot-ic-uh]
"I get this *exotica* leg pain when I dance."
See also: *skyattic*

Fibermylasha   Fibromyalgia
[fahy-ber-mahy-lash-uh]
"I saw the TV commercial…I think I have *fibermylasha*."
See also: *fibernailasha*

Fibernailasha   Fibromyalgia
[fahy-ber-nail-ash-uh]
"I have pain. Can I get the test for *fibernailasha*?"
See also: *fibermylasha*

Fireball   Fibroid
[fahy-er-bawl]
"There are *fireballs* in my uterus"

Hepatitis 3   Hepatitis C
[hep-uh-tahy-tus three]
"My liver is sick with *hepatitis 3*"

Herny   Hernia
[her-nee]
"The *herny* shot out when I lifted the refrigerator."
See also: *hyena*

High anal hernia   Hiatal hernia
[hahy ey-nyl hur-nee-uh]
"I always get *gas reflux* from my *high anal hernia*."

Hyena   Hernia
[hahy-ee-nuh]
"I have a *hyena* in my groin."
See also: *herny*

Independicitis   Appendicitis
[in-di-pen-duh-cytus]
"The stomach pain must be *independicitis.*"

Infant tango   Impetigo
[in-fuhnt tang-oh]
"My baby had the *infant tango*."
See also: *infatigo*

Infatigo   Impetigo
[in-fah-tye-go]
"I used some skin cream for the *infatigo*."
See also: *infant tango*

Intoxidicated   Intoxicated
[in-tok-si-da-kay-tid]
"I only had only two beers, I am not *intoxidicated*!"

Irresistible bowel   Irritable bowel
syndrome   syndrome
[ir-ee-zis-tuh-buhl bou-ul]
"Oh no, my *irresistible bowel syndrome* is acting up."

John Stevens   Stevens Johnson syndrome

[jon stee-vuhns]

"I got a bad rash and they sent me to the burn ward with *John Stevens*."

Lucas   Lupus

[loo-kuhs]

"My legs hurt. I think I'm having a *lucas* flare."

Lung mask   Lung mass

[luhng mask]

"They may have seen a *lung mask* on the x-ray."

Magnum degeneration   Macular degeneration

[mag-nuhm de-jen-uh-rey-shun]

"The *magnum degeneration* makes it hard to see."

Micro valve prolap   Mitral valve prolapse

[mahy-kroh valv proh-lap]

"The *micro valve prolap* gives me heart *palpations*."

Migrant   Migraine
[mahy-grunt]
"This headache is bad, it must be a *migrant*."

Missed carriage   Miscarriage
[misd kar-ij]
"The doctors can't find the baby, they think it *missed carriage*."

Mullet finger   Mallet finger
[muhl-lit fing-ger]
"Hey Ma, doc says I got a *mullet finger*…wanna see?"

OCPD   COPD
[o.c.p.d]
"I needed extra *albooterall* today for my *OCPD*."

Old timer's   Alzheimers
[ohld-tymers]
"My grandfather has *old timer's* disease."

Oscar cirrhosis   Osteoporosis
[os-ker si-roh-sis]
"My bones are brittle from *oscar cirrhosis*."

Otus media   Otitis media
[oh-tus me-dee-uh]
"At least its only *otus media*, I was afraid he had an ear infection."

Pollinated cyst   Pilonidal cyst
[pol-luh-nay-ted sist]
"I think the *spider bite* gave me a *pollinated cyst*."

Polp   Polyp
[puhlp]
"They saw *polps* on the colonoscopy."

POS   PCOS
[p.o.s.]
"The doc thinks my irregular periods and facial hair are from *POS*."

Prophylactic   Anaphylactic
shock   shock

[proh-fuh-lak-tik shok]

"I got stung by a bee and went into *prophylactic shock*."

Robomalitis   Osteomyelitis

[roh-bo-mahl-ey-tus]

"I was on an antibiotic for bone *robomalitis*."

Scardosis   Sarcoidosis

[skahr-doh-sis]

"The cough is from *scardosis*."

Second degree   Secondary
infection   infection

[sek-uhnd duh-gree]

"First I had a cold, now the doctor says I have a bacterial *second degree infection*."

Septitz   Sepsis

[sep-tits]

"I was in the hospital for a *septitz* infection."

Skyattic   Sciatic nerve
[skahy-at-ik]
"The pain is from up in my *skyattic* nerves."
See also: *exotica*

Sleep acnea   Sleep apnea
[sleep ak-nee-uh]
"I wear a machine at night to clear up my *sleep acnea*."

Stationary   Gestational
diabetes   diabetes
[stay-shun-ner-ee dahy-uh-bee-teez]
"I stayed in bed when I was pregnant and got *stationary diabetes*."

Sick as hell   Sickle cell
anemia   anemia
[sik az hel uh-nee-mee-uh]
"I've got a history of *sick as hell anemia*."

Sinkapeed   Syncope
[sink-uh-peeyd]
"The doctor said I passed out and *sinkapeed* myself."

Silosis   Scoliosis
[sahy-lo-sys]
"My spine got bent by *silosis*."

Spinal espinosis   Spinal stenosis
[spahyn-el ez-pin-oh-sis]
"The *spinal espinosis* is always painful."

Split dick   Slipped disk
[split dik]
"The MRI showed a *split dick* and *spinal espinosis*."

Stripped throat   Strep throat
[stript throht]
"It's hard to swallow with this *stripped throat*."

Tacardia   Tachycardia
[tuh-kahr-dee-uh]
"I have a history of heart *populations* and *tacardia*."

Tenderitis   Tendonitis
[ten-duhr-ey-tus]
"My wrist hurts, I think its *tenderitis*."

Thrust   Thrush
[thruhst]
"I think my baby got *thrust* in his mouth."

Track infection   Urinary tract infection
[trak in-fek-shuhn]
"I keep running to the bathroom, I must have a *track infection*."

Unstitchable cystitis   Interstitial cystitis
[un-stich-uh-bal sis-tye-tus]
"My bladder problem can't be fixed, its *unstitchable cystitis*."

Uppertory respertery infection   Upper respiratory
[uhp-er-tohr-ee res-per-tehry]
"I'm on these antibiotics for some *uppertory respertery infection*."

Verticalosis   Diverticulosis
[vur-ti-kuhl-oh-sis]
"The colonoscopy showed bowel *verticalosis*."

Very close veins   Varicose veins
[ver-ee klohz veinz]
"Look at these *very close veins* on the surface my legs."

Vitatagleo   Vitiligo
[vee-tuh-tag-leo]
"Do I have that Michael Jackson disease, *vitatagleo*?"

Wing worm   Tinea capitis
[wing wurm]
"He takes medicine for *wing worm* on the head."

Layman's Terms:

Medications

"Doc, I need a subscription for…"

Actos   Altace
[ak-tos]
"I don't have diabetes. I take the *actos* for blood pressure."
See also: *all taste*

Acktoast   Actos
[ak-tohst]
"I eat the *acktoast* for my *sugar*."

Albitaroll   Albuterol
[al-bit-uh-rohl]
"The *albitaroll* helps my *breevin*."
See also: *albooterall, al-brutal*

Albooterall   Albuterol
[al-boo-ter-rawl]
"My asthma is better thanks to *albooterall*."
See also: *albitaroll, al-brutal*

Al-brutal   Albuterol
[al-broo-tuhl]
"I had to use the *al-brutal* puffer for my asthma."
See also: *albitaroll*

All taste   Altace
[awl teyst]
"I'm on *all taste* for my *high blood*."
See also: *actos*

Amy Tripoli   Amitriptyline
[ey-mee trip-oh-lee]
"I've felt great ever since I got on *Amy Tripoli*."

Anniebiotics   Antibiotics
[an-ee-bahy-yo-tiks]
"I got a really bad cold, I need some *anniebiotics*."

Appendix shot   Tetanus shot
[uh-pen-diks shot]
"My arm really hurts from the *appendix shot*."
See also: *technitz shot, tetanus shop, texas shot*

Bapository   Suppository
[buh-pah-zeh-tor-ree]
"You want me to do WHAT with the *bapository*?"
See also: *depository, pository, suppositers*

Bassyum   Potassium
[bas-see-um]
"I started the *bassyum* after my *electric lights* were off."

Bin Laden   Dilaudid
[bin lah-den]
"Motrin ain't workin, I need *Bin Laden*!"
See also: *dilada, dilaunten, dilaudy, dillahdid, diluted*

Clavitz   Plavix
[clah-vits]
"I've been on *clavitz* since my heart attack."

Clonidine   Klonopin
[kloh-ni-deen]
"He takes *clonidine* 0.5 for his *nerves*."

Coudamin   Coumadin
[cooh-dah-min]
"I take *coudamin* for *thick blood*."

Depository   Suppository
[dee-po-zeh-tor-ree]
"Eww, I ain't using no *depository*, that's a one-way street."
See also: *bapository, pository, suppositers*

Dilada   Dilaudid
[di-lah-da]
"I need *dilada* when my *fibermylasha* gets bad."
See also: *Bin Laden, dilaunten, dilaudy, dillahdid, diluted*

Dilaunten   Dilaudid
[di-lawn-ten]
"Uhh, it started with a 'D'…umm, I think it was *dilaunten*."
See also: *Bin Laden, dilada, dilaudy, dillahdid, diluted*

Dilaudy   Dilaudid
[di-law-dee]
"I'm allergic to everything, except *dilaudy*…"
See also: *Bin Laden, dilada, dilaunten, dillahdid, diluted*

Dillahdid _____ Dilaudid

[dil-lahh-did]

"I need 3mg of *dillahdid* and *subscription* for *percs*!"

See also: *Bin Laden, dilada, dilaunten, dilaudy, diluted*

Diluted _____ Dilaudid

[di-loo-ted]

"The *diluted* is the only thing that works for my pain."

See also: *Bin Laden, dilada, dilaunten, dillahdid, dilaudy*

Dioxin _____ Digoxin

[dahy-ok-sin]

"I take the *dioxin* for my a-fib."

Fenagin _____ Phenergan

[fen-uh-gin]

"My *vomicking* stopped after the *fenagin*."

Fraternity pills _____ Fertility pills

[frah-tur-ni-tee pilz]

"I wanna have a kid so I'm takin' the *fraternity pills*."

See also: *baby pills*

Flem-torr   Antiinflammatory

[flem tor]

"The *flem-torr* medicine didn't work for my back pain."

Flexo fenadreen   Fexofenadine

[flex-oh fen-nuh-dreen]

"My allergies are much better with the *flexo fenadreen*."

Flomax   Flonase

[floh-max]

"When I get a runny nose I use my *flomax*."

Genericer   Generic

[juh-ner-ri-ker]

"I need the real medicine, the *genericer* don't work for me."

Glucafog   Glucophage

[glue-kuh-fog]

"The *glucafog* helps my *sugar*."

Holidall   Haldol
[hah-lee-dawl]
"I'm allergic to *holidall*…"

Hydrochloride   Hydrochlorothiazide
[hahy-droh-klaw-rahyd]
"The *hydrochloride* helps my *high blood*."

Ibreproferen   Ibuprofen
[ahy-bree-pro-fuhr-rin]
"I'm *eating ibreproferens* like candy, I need something stronger."

In da medicine   Indomethacin
[in da me-duh-sin]
"*In da medicine* helps with my gout pains."

Inflammatory   Antiinflammatory
[in-flam-uh-taw-ree]
"I've been using an *inflammatory* to help with the swelling."

Latex   Lasix
[lay-tex]
"My legs was *swold* so they *subscribed latex* pills."

Loonexa   Lunesta
[loo-nex-uh]
"*Loonexa* helps me sleep."

Mayfromen   Metformin
[may-fro-mun]
"The *mayfromen* is for my *sugar*."

Mo-train   Motrin
[moh-treyn]
"The *mo-trains* don't work for my pains."

Moxcillin   Amoxicillin
[mock-sil-len]
"Can I get some *moxcillin* for my cold?"

My-sins   Macrolide "mycin" Abx
[mahy sinz]
"I'm allergic to *my-sins*."

Nappyum   Naprosyn
[nah-pee-yum]
"I'm allergic to *nappyum* and tramadol."

Narcons   Narcan
[nar-kohns]
"Why'd you give me *narcons*!?? You owe me four bags of heroin!"

Near sporen   Neosporin
[neer spor-ren]
"I've been using *near sporen* around the cut."

Neck seen   Nexium
[nek seen]
"I take *neck seen* for my *gas reflux*."

New rotten .... Neurontin
[noo rot-ten]
"I tried *new rotten* for the *fibermylasha* pain."

Oxy-cotton .... Oxycontin
[ok-see kot-ten]
"I ate some of my mom's *oxy-cotton* to help with my *toof* pain."

Pellesillium .... Penicillin
[pel-luh-sil-lee-um]
"I took some of my baby's left over *pellesillium*..."

Pository .... Suppository
[poh-zeh-tor-ree]
"The tylenol *pository* took away the fevers."
See also: *bapository, depository, suppositers*

Raglin .... Reglan
[rag-lyn]
"I usually take *raglin* for my *migrants*."

Silmitifen   Acetaminophen
[sil-meh-teh-fen]
"I gave my baby a *silmitifen bapository* for the fever."

Silver cream   Silvadene
[sil-ver kreem]
"He's been using *silver cream* on the burns."

Sipatory   Lipitor
[si-puh-tohr-ee]
"I take *sipatory* for my cholesterol."

Spyvera   Spiriva
[spahy-vee-ruh]
"My breathing is better with the *spyvera puffer*."

Stemofastic   Simvastatin
[steh-moh-faz-tek]
"I take *stemofastic* for cholesterol."

Subscription   Prescription
[sub-skrip-shun]
"My *subscription* for *oxy-cotton* ran out, can I get a new one?"

Sulfur   Sulfa
[suhl-fer]
"I'm allergic to *sulfur*, *pellesillium*, *my-sins...*"

Suppositers   Suppository
[suh-poz-zih-ters]
"I like *suppositers*, they help my constipation."
See also: *bapository*, *depository*, *pository*

Technitz shot   Tetanus shot
[tek-nytz shot]
"I got a *technitz shot* when I got stitches last year."
See also: *appendix shot*, *tetanus shop*, *texas shot*

Tetanus shop   Tetanus shot
[tet-nuhs shop]
"I stepped on a nail and I'm looking for a *tetanus shop*."
See also: *appendix shot*, *technitz shot*, *texas shot*

Texas shot   Tetanus shot
[tek-sus shot]
"I got a *texas shot* after I cut my hand at the Alamo."
See also: *appendix shot, technitz shot, tetanus shop*

Tie in all   Tylenol
[tahy in awl]
"The fevers came down after *tie in all*."

Toe pull   Toprol
[toh-puhl]
"The *toe pull* is for my heart."

Well bootin'   Wellbutrin
[wel boot-en]
"I been pukin' since I started *well bootin*"

Layman's Terms:

Procedures

Wait, you're gonna do what now?

Boob transplants   Breast implants
[boob trans-plahnt]
"My friend got *boob transplants* and I want some too!"

Cabbage   CABG / bypass
[kab-ij]
"Wait doc, are you saying I can only eat *cabbage* after my heart bypass?"

Cat skin   CAT (CT) scan
[kat skin]
"Eww, I ain't drinkin' no *cat skin* prep!"

Circle-cision   Circumcision
[sur-kuhl sih-zuhn]
"My son ain't getting a *circle-cision*! It might get cut off!"

Colonoffapee   Colonoscopy
[koh-luhn-of-fuh-pee]
"Hello, I'm here for my *colonoffapee*."
See also: *colonossofy, columnopstopy, columnostopy*

Colonossofy   Colonoscopy
[koh-luhn-nos-suh-fee]
"My *colonossofy* found some polyps."
See also: *colonoffapee, columnopstopy, columnostopy*

Colostomy   Colposcopy
[kuhl-os-tuh-mee]
"The gynecologist did a *colostomy* to check my cervix."

Columnopstopy   Colonoscopy
[koh-luhm-nop-sto-pee]
"For my 50th birthday the doctor gave me a *columnopstopy*."
See also: *colonoffapee, colonossofy, columnostopy*

Columnostopy   Colonoscopy
[kol-uhm-os-toh-pee]
"For the *columnostopy*, you put that thing where?!"
See also: *colonoffapee, colonossofy, columnopstopy*

Enscopy   Endoscopy
[en-skuh-pee]
"They saw a *high anal hernia* with the *enscopy*."

Fibulizer   Defibrillator
[fib-yoo-lahy-zer]
"The doctor planted a *fibulizer* in my chest."

Folotomy   Phlebotomy
[ful-lah-tuh-mee]
"I'm learning to draw blood in *folotomy* school."

Histerackme   Hysterectomy
[his-tuh-rak-mee]
"I was passing *clogs* for months so I got a *histerackme*."

Histerossofy   Hysteroscopy
[his-ter-ros-suh-fee]
"My gynecologist checked me with a *histerossofy*."

Incubated   Intubated
[ink-yoo-bey-ted]
"Her baby was *incubated* for bad breathing."
See also: *Inkabated*

Inkabated   Intubated
[ink-uh-bey-ted]
"My asthma was so bad I had to get *inkabated*."
See also: *Incubated*

Labia repair   Labral repair
[ley-bee-uh ree-pair]
"This shoulder really hurts. They said I need a *labia repair*."

Lobotomy   Laparotomy
[luh-buh-tuh-mee]
"My abdominal pains were so bad they had to do an exploratory *lobotomy*."

MIR   MRI
[M.I.R.]
"Here's the *MIR* report for my *lumbex disco* bulge."

Place-maker   Pacemaker
[plays-mey-ker]
"My heart stopped working, so they put in a *place-maker*."

Radio-ology   Radiology
[rey-dee-oh oh-luh-jee]
"They're sending me to *radio-ology* for some sort of *cat skin*."

Sensarian   Cesarean
section   section
[sen-ser-ree-un sek-shun]
"The labor hurt so bad they had to do a *sensarian section*."
See also: *serious section*

Serious   Cesarean
section   section
[seer-ree-uhs sek-shun]
"The baby wouldn't come out, so I needed a *serious section*."
See also: *sensarian section*

Stem   Stent
[stem]
"The cardiologist put in a *stem* after my heart attack."
See also: *stint*

Stint   Stent

[stint]

"I needed a *stint* because of the chest pain."

See also: *stem*

Tubalation   Tubal ligation

[too-buhl-lay-shun]

"They did my *tubalation* after the *serious section*."

See also: *tubalization, tubal litigation*

Tubalization   Tubal ligation

[too-buh-lahy-zay-shun]

"I got a *tubalization* after my eighth child was born."

See also: *tubalation, tubal litigation*

Tubal litigation   Tubal ligation

[too-buhl lit-i-gey-shun]

"I can't be pregnant. I had a *tubal litigation*…I'm calling my lawyer!"

See also: *tubalation, tubalization*

Upadural   Epidural
[up-uh-duhr-rel]
"I got an *upadural* before my *serious section*."

Urinology   Urinalysis
[yoor-in-ol-luh-jee]
"They're checking my pee with *urinology*."

Layman's Terms:

Terms That Defy Categorization

I just don't know…

Ambalance   Ambulance

[am-bah-luhns]

"I found a tick on my arm so I called the *ambalance*."

Carpractor   Chiropractor

[kar-prak-ter]

"The *carpractor* helped my back pain after the accident."

Club sierra   Klebsiella

[klub see-ur-ruh]

"I was on antibiotics for *club sierra* ammonia."

Compacted   Impacted

[kom-pak-ted]

"I got *compacted* wisdom teeth. Tylenol ain't been workin."

Congenial   Congenital

[kuhn-jee-ny-uhl]

"My baby had *congenial* heart problems."

Death   Deaf
[deth]
"The music was so loud I think I'm *death*."

Electric lights   Electrolytes
[il-lek-trik lahyts]
"I don't feel good 'cause my *electric lights* are off."

Family position   Family physician
[fah-muh-lee puh-zi-shuhn]
"I know. I know…I need to get me a *family position*."

Festation   Infestation
[fes-tey-shun]
"It itches *down there*…I think I got a crab *festation*."

Groinocologist   Gynecologist
[groy-ni-kol-uh-jist]
"The *groinocologist* checked my cervix."

Halter monitor   Holter monitor
[hawl-ter mo-neh-ter]
"I shouldn't have worn a halter top with the *halter monitor*."

Horspital   Hospital
[hawrs-pi-tl]
"The donkey bit me, so I came to the *horspital*."

Helf   Health
[helf]
"The dentist said I got bad *toof helf*."

Hemaglaben   Hemoglobin
[hee-muh-gloh-ben]
"I'm *anemix* from low blood *hemaglaben*."

Hemacratene   Hematocrit
[hee-ma-krah-teh-nee]
"My *hemaglaben* and *hemacratene* were low last month."

Hillin   Healing
[hil-len]
"The boil ain't <u>*hillin*</u>."

Hopkiss   Hospice
[hop-kis]
"They took him off <u>*hopkiss*</u> because he didn't die."

Libido   Equilibrium
[li-bee-doh]
"My father can't walk straight. His <u>*libido*</u> is all off."

Magnet   Maggot
[mag-nit]
"This wound ain't *hillin*. Can I use <u>*magnets*</u> in it?"

Mercer   MRSA
[muhr-sir]
"My girlfriend has the <u>*mercer*</u> and I'd like to be checked
for it too."
See also: *mercy, moosra*

Mercy   MRSA
[mur-see]
"I picked up the *mercy* infections from jail."
See also: *mercer, moosra*

Moosra   MRSA
[moos-rah]
"I thought it was a *spider bite*, but it was really the *moosra*."
See also: *mercer, mercy*

Narcrotic   Narcotic
[nar-cro-tic]
"But I need a *narcrotic*, this paper-cut hurts really bad."

Nervologist   Neurologist
[nur-vo-luh-jist]
"I'm scheduled to see a *nervologist* for my foot tingling."

Pediatric award   Pediatric ward
[pee-dee-ah-trik uh-wawrd]
"My son got sent to the *pediatric award*."

Percussions   Compressions
[per-kuh-shuhnz]
"I learned *percussions* in CPR class."

Physician's   Physician
apprentice   assistant
[fi-zi-shuns uh-pren-tis]
"The *physician's apprentice* said my ankle was broke."

Pullomerry   Pulmonary
[pul-loh-meh-ree]
"The *pullomery* disease makes it hard to *breeve*."

Scavies   Scabies
[skay-vees]
"There's no way I have *scavies*! It's probably just crabs, again."

Seduce   Sedate
[si-doos]
"The doctor *seduced* me to fix my broken arm."

Slint   Sling or Splint
[slint]
"I've been wearing the *slint* since I broke my elbow."

Sterilate   Sterilize
[steh-ri-late]
"It's infected? But I *sterilated* the needle by soaking it in beer…"

Submit   Admit / Commit
[suhb-mit]
"Hello, my wife is crazy and I'd like to *submit* her."

Suffercate   Suffocate
[suh-fer-keyt]
"He can't take a *bref*! I think he's gonna *suffercate*!"

Triglyceroids   Triglycerides
[tri-gly-suh-roids]
"My *triglyceroids* are really high."

Vowel	Bowel
movement	movement

[vow-uhl mov-muhnt]

"It hurts down there when I have a *vowel movement*."

Layman's Terms:

Laypersons' Medical Slang

"Doc…spare me your medical mumbo jumbo!"
- Homer Simpson

Agita   Indigestion

[ah-ji-tuh]

"Hot peppers give me *agita*."

Ammonia in my liver   Hepatitis

[uh-mohn-yuh]

"The blood tests showed *ammonia in my liver*"

Arthur   Arthritis

[ahr-ther]

"I've known *Arthur* for years. He gives me pain, I give him motrin."

Baby pills   Fertility pills

[bey-bee pilz]

"I'm taking *baby pills* so I can have me a baby."

See also: *fraternity pills*

Burned   Contracted an STD

[burnd]

"I slept with some girl last month and I think I got *burned*."

Changed life   Underwent menopause

[cheynjd lyfe]

"I've had hot flashes ever since I *changed life*."

Cold knife scraping   D&C procedure

[kohld nahyf skrey-peng]

"After months of vaginal bleeding, they did a *cold knife scraping*."

Cold in my kidney   Pyelonephritis

[kohld in mahy kid-nee]

"I'm taking antibiotics for fever and *cold in my kidney*."

Consumption   Tuberculosis

[kuhn-suhmp-shuhn]

"My son has been coughing. I think he's got *consumption*."

See also: *red snapper*

Coughing up   Expectorating
cold   sputum

[kawf-ing uhp kohld]

"I been *coughing up cold* all day. I need an antibiotic."

| Degenerative tooth disease | Chronic tooth decay |

[dee-jen-ner-ruh-tiv tooth di-zeez]
"The *degenerative tooth disease* runs in my family."

| Done fell out | Loss of consciousness |

[duhn fel out]
"That boy drank too much beer and *done fell out*."
See also: *fell out*

| Down there | Reference to the genitals |

[doun ther]
"I…uhh…have a lump…*down there* [motioning downward]."

| Eat | Take medication PO |

[eet]
"I been *eating* motrin all day…the only thing that works is the *percs*."

Fell out   Loss of consciousness
[fel out]
"Well doc, I stood up and then I fell out."
See also: *done fell out*

Fever   Redness & swelling
[fee-ver]
"It looks like this bug bite is *swold* and getting a *fever*."

Flow   Menstrual period
[floh]
"My *flow* is so heavy this month. I'm passing *clogs*!"
See also: *monthly*

Fluid ran over-full   Polyhydramnios
[floo-id ran oh-ver ful]
"My OB/GYN doctor was worried my *fluid ran over-full*."

Hair bumps   Folliculitis
[air bumpz]
"I was in the hot tub, now I got me some *hair bumps*."

High five   HIV

[hi fahyv]

"I know I got *the clap*. Can you also check me for the *high five*?"

Kidney   Acute

collapse   renal failure

[kid-nee kuh-laps]

"The doctor said I might need dialysis because my *kidneys collapsed*."

Monthly   Menstrual period

[muhnth-lee]

"I need a pregnancy test. My *monthly* got skipped."

See also: *flow*

Mune   Mucus

[myoon]

"I've been coughing up *mune* all week."

Nerves   Any psych issue

[nurvz]

"My friend got put in the psych-ward for his *nerves*."

Percs   Percocet
[perks]
"Hey man, I got the *percs*. You got the money?"

Pharming   Obtaining Rx drugs
[fahr-ming]
"I did some *pharming* at my granny's house and found a few *percs*."

Piles   Hemorrhoids
[pahylz]
"I got big hard *piles*. Sometimes they bleed when I pinch a loaf."

Puffer   Inhaler
[puhf-fer]
"I'm wheezing and I can't find my *puffer*."

Pus bag   Abscess or Boil
[puhs bag]
"Dude, you gotta see the huge *pus bag* from that *spider bite*!"
See also: *absets, absence, ass cyst, risen, spider bite*

Pussed out   Drained pus

[puhst out]

"My abscess got all swollen and then *pussed out*."

Pussing   To extrude pus

[puhs-en]

"This boil is *pussing* out nasty."

Raw   Painful

[raw]

"My thumb is feeling all *raw* since it got hit with a hammer."

Red snapper   Tuberculosis

[red snap-per]

"This cough won't stop. I think I got the *red snapper*."

See also: *consumption*

Risen   Abscess or Boil

[rayh-zuhn]

"I think I have a *risen* on my leg. It's all *raw* and has a *fever*."

See also: *absets, absence, ass cyst, pus bag, spider bite*

Spider bite   Abscess or Boil
[spahy-der byte]
"No, I didn't see a spider, but its gotta be an infected *spider bite*."
See also: *absets, absence, ass cyst, pus bag, risen*

Stepmother   Hangnail
[step-muh-ther]
"I tried to pull the *stepmother* off my finger. Now it's bleeding."

Sugar   Diabetes
[shoo-ger]
"My grandma's got *sugar*. She takes shots for it."

Sugar pill   Diabetes medication
[shoo-ger pil]
"I take *sugar pills* for my *sugar*-diabetes."

The clamity   Cold & clammy
[thuh klam-uh-tee]
"Cold and sweaty? Yeah, I got *the clamity*."

The clap   Gonorrhea

[thuh klap]

"I got the tap, now I got *the clap*…"

Totem pole   Xanax 2mg

[toh-tuhm pohl]

"Hey man, can I trade a *totem pole* for two *percs*?"

See also: *zaneeze*

Tropical   Topical

[truh-pi-kuhl]

This rash just isn't getting better with the *tropical* steroids.

Vikes   Vicodin

[vhyks]

"Can I get some *Percs*? The *Vikes* don't work for me…"

Water   Edema

[wah-ter]

"The *water-pill* gets rid of the *water* in my legs."

Water on the heart	Congestive heart failure

[wah-ter on thuh hahrt]

"I take two *latex* pills for *water on the heart*."

Zaneeze	Xanax

[zay-nees]

"Can I get an order of *zaneeze* and a large *perc* to go?"

See also: *totem pole*

Blood-related issues:

High blood	Hypertension

[hahy bluhd]

"I take lisinopril for *high blood*."

Low blood	Anemia

[loh bluhd]

"I take iron pills for *low blood*."

Thin blood	Coagulopathy

[thin bluhd]

"My Coumadin level showed *thin blood*."

Thick blood   Hypercoagulability
[thik bluhd]
"I take *coudamin* 'cause I got *thick blood*."

Layman's Terms:

Clinicians' Medical Slang

Just a random sampling…

Antibioticise   Start antibiotics
[an-ti-bahy-yoh-ti-sahyz]
"Mr. Smith has pneumonia. I'll *antibioticise* him."

Blomit   Blood in vomit
[blah-mit]
"The patient is a 60 year old male on warfarin with nausea and *blomiting*."

Brutain   Physical restraint
[bru-tayhn]
"The placement of sutures was facilitated by a mild dose of brutain."

Cheeto Sign   Clinical indicator*
[cheeh-toh sahyn]
"Patient reports vomiting. Positive *Cheeto sign* noted on exam."
* See "Definitions" chapter

Earrigation   Irrigation of ear
[eer-ri-gehy-shun]
"The cerumen was removed with *earrigation*."

Herpeschlonger   Male w/genital herpes
[hur-peez-shlong-gur]
"25 year old *herpeschlonger* needs acyclovir refill."

Incarceritis   Post-arrest illness
[in-kahr-ser-ri-tis]
"He was arrested then developed acute *incarceritis*."

Metabolizing to Freedom   Awaiting sobriety*
[muh-tah-buh-lahy-zing]
"He had an alcohol of 627. He's now awake and *metabolizing to freedom*."
* See "Definitions" chapter

O-sign   Clinical indicator*
[oh-sahyn]
"Patient sleeping, *O-sign* noted, patient placed on supplemental O2."
* See "Definitions" chapter

Q-sign   Clinical indicator*
[kyoo-sahyn]
"No improvement with oxygen. *O-sign* has progressed to
Q-sign, rapid response team notified."
* See "Definitions" chapter

Sewage soak   Iodine wound soaking*
[soo-ij sohk]
"Please remove his hand from the *sewage soak* and irrigate
the wound."
* See "Definitions" chapter

Suitcase sign   Clinical indicator*
[soot-kehys sahyn]
"Patient arrived via EMS with a mild COPD exacerbation,
exhibiting a positive *suitcase sign*."
* See "Definitions" chapter

The Dwindles   Age-related decline
[the dwin-dlz]
"The 95 year old gentleman is slowly dying of *the
dwindles*."

Layman's Terms:

Written Words

*It's amazing what you'll find on a chart or medical
history sheet*

Written word:	Interpretation:
"Adapost"	Adipose
"Anklososin spinulosis"	Ankylosing spondylosis
"Arotic aneurysm"	Aortic aneurysm
"Atacacardia svt"	A tachycardia: SVT
"Atalexitatis"	Atelectasis
"Breast modules"	Breast nodules
"Cabbage"	CABG

Written word:	Interpretation:
"Corpal tunnel"	Carpal tunnel
"Dimension"	Dementia
"Diverticulities"	"Diverticulitis"
"Ematrex"	Imitrex
"Endescope"	Endoscopy
"Eptopic pregnancy"	Ectopic pregnancy
"Frendectomy"	Frenulotomy

Written word:	Interpretation:
"H_2O 25mg"	Unknown?
"High Pertension"	Hypertension
"Hypostatic hypotension"	Orthostatic hypotension
"Impression"	Compression
"Intoxification"	Intoxication
"Allergy: Lactaid"	Lactose
"Laprascoptomy"	Laparoscopy

Written word:	Interpretation:
"Line titer"	Lyme titer
"Minnie stroke"	Mini-stroke (TIA)
"Mofeen"	Morphine
"Munshinghowsens"	Munchausen's disease
"Patent dutus arterisus"	Patent ductus arteriosus
"Polinitol cyst"	Pilonidal cyst
"Pyanodal cyst"	Pilonidal cyst

Written word:	Interpretation:
"Porkacet"	Percocet
"Prayer: full strength"	Bayer: full strength
"Rotocuff"	Rotator cuff
"Short guy syndrome"	Short bowel syndrome
"Sueda"	Seizure
"Swellon"	Swollen
"Thrust"	Thrush

Written word:	Interpretation:
"Tubligation"	Tubal ligation
"Uterisstillin"	Uterus is still in
"Varisies of Osophogus"	Esophageal Varices
"Verikoseal"	Varicocele

Layman's Terms:

Definitions

*These definitions might not be accurate but
I thought they were fun.
(For entertainment purposes only. Not for
actual clinical use.)*

Clinical Indicator:

Term:
Cheeto Sign

Definition:
The "Cheeto sign" refers to the physical exam finding of cheese-dust on the patient's hands and/or mouth area. This clinical indicator is used to assess the acuity of a patient complaining of nausea, vomiting, abdominal pain, or dysphagia. Since most emergency department waiting rooms have a vending machine stocked with the irresistible snack, the Cheeto sign is surprisingly accurate.

Consider a typical scenario in which the Cheeto sign is helpful: A patient reports "I keep throwing up and can't keep anything down." A quick glance around the examination room reveals several empty bags of cheese doodles, with doodle remnants noted around the patient's mouth. This constitutes a "positive" Cheeto sign. (A positive finding can be further evaluated with the Cheese-Dust Score on the following page.)

In contrast, a "negative" Cheeto sign would be reported in a patient with direct access to the delicious snack food and without cheese-dust on the hands or face, provided that (1) The patient has not washed his/her hands or face and (2) The patient is not allergic to cheesy-goodness.

Disclaimer (as recommended by our legal counsel): The above mentioned "Cheeto Sign" is in no way affiliated with the popular cheesy snack Cheetos®, a registered trademark of Frito-Lay. In addition, any other trademark, product, or business that may have been mentioned elsewhere in this book has absolutely no connection, affiliation, or relationship with this book whatsoever.

Clinical Indicator:

Term:
Cheese-Dust Score

To further quantify the value of the doodle, we introduce the Cheese-Dust Score (CDS). Upon the determination of a positive Cheeto sign, the CDS may be employed. The CDS is a simple test that assigns points based on cheese-dust findings by physical exam:

+1—Cheese-dust localized to dominant hand and/or lips
+1—Cheese-dust on bilateral hands
+1—Cheese-dust on face and/or front of shirt/gown
+2—Cheese-dust in hair or rear of shirt/gown
+2—Patient chomping on doodles during the exam
-2—Physical exam (with distraction) consistent with complaint (e.g. abdominal tenderness or dry heaves)
-2—Patient vomits on self and/or examiner

The CDS score is inversely proportional to the patient's acuity, based on the following table:

Score 5-6+ = Low index of concern
Score 2-4 = Moderate index of concern
Score <2 = High index of concern

Term:
McDonald's Medicine

Definition:
The form of medicine in which patient care is expected with the speed of a drive-thru window. Because of today's expectations of instant service, immediate gratification, and a hot bacon-double-cheeseburger in 60 seconds or less, it is no wonder that some patients have come to demand the same service from their medical providers.

To fully understand the phenomenon of McDonald's Medicine (or "McMed") we'll use a hypothetical patient in an emergency department. To be fully satisfied a McMed patient should receive the following:

- Access to a medical provider within seconds of arriving
- Have the ability to provide a list of problems, some dating back several decades
- Be provided with *the* pill that will immediately cure every problem and have no side effects
- Be given the opportunity to order additional medications, as desired (e.g. "2 percs, 1 zanee, and a vike to go, please")
- Have every problem diagnosed, treated, and cured in 30 minutes or less
- Receive a complementary order of "large fries and a *diet* coke" upon hospital discharge

Note: The terms "McDonald's Medicine" & "McMed" have no affiliation with the popular fast-food chain that promptly delivers greasy-goodness in a burger-shaped patty of delicious atherosclerotic obesity. Yummy.

Term:
Metabolizing to Freedom (MTF)

Definition:
Highly intoxicated people are often brought to the emergency department to get checked out. Although this may be appropriate if the intoxicated patient is hardly breathing, in many cases the patient is brought in just to "sleep it off." Because of legal concerns, the intoxicated patient is typically kept in the ER until s/he is sober or until a friend/family member agrees to take responsibility for a mildly intoxicated patient. Depending on the patient's alcohol level, this stay in the ER can last anywhere from a couple of hours to several weeks (seemingly...). During this waiting time, the patient is effectively in an alcohol-induced limbo and is considered to be "Metabolizing to Freedom."

Clinical Indicator:

Term:
O-Sign

Definition:
The "O-Sign" refers to the circular O-like shape a patient's mouth forms when he or she is unconscious or deeply sleeping. As muscle tone decreases the patient's mouth often opens into an increasingly wider "O". When paired with a measurement of the patient's respiratory rate, the O-sign can be used to determine a patient's relative stability. While the O-sign is usually reported as positive or negative, the value of the O-sign can be further increased by including an O-sign diameter measurement. The diameter measurement should reflect the distance (in centimeters) between the top and bottom lips when an O-sign is found to be present.

A patient typically becomes less stable as the O-sign diameter increases and respiratory rate decreases. Thus, the O-sign diameter might be helpful as an additional vital sign.

Clinical Indicator:

Term:
Q-sign

Definition:
Similar to the previously mentioned O-sign, the "Q-sign" reflects a patient's relative stability and ability to control his or her own airway. Unconsciousness or deep sleep is usually accompanied by a decrease in muscle tone. As muscle tone decreases the mouth often opens (positive O-sign) and sometimes culminates in the manifestation of a positive Q-sign. The Q-sign is considered positive when a patient's tongue flops outward beyond the open lips, giving the appearance of the letter "Q".

In most cases, the development of a Q-sign should be considered an ominous finding.

Term:
Sewage Soak

Definition:
There are many ways to clean out a laceration or wound. One frequently used (although inappropriate) method to clean a hand or foot wound is to pour Betadine and water into a basin and allow the injured appendage to soak. This method successfully turns the skin a wonderful shade of orange, but does little to actually clean the wound. As an added benefit, prolonged soaking of the wound-area typically causes the surrounding skin to shrivel (like a raisin) into a friable orange-colored mess, making suturing the area more difficult. Due to the relative ineffectiveness of soaking a wound in a stagnant pool of Betadine, and because of the actual appearance of Betadine in a basin, this method of wound cleaning has been termed a "Sewage Soak".

Note: Please do not actually use this method. Irrigation with sterile saline or water is both more effective and less staining (especially if splashed on your clean white coat).

(Betadine®, Purdue Products L.P., is a spectacular product if used as intended, on intact skin or very superficial wounds…not poured deep into a wound crevice.)

Term:
Spider Bite

Definition:
Any abnormal swollen red spot on the skin, typically without a known cause. This term is commonly used when describing an area of the skin that is red, inflamed, and painful. Most "spider bite" victims self-diagnose this affliction, usually with the input of their most medically-inclined friend or family member (example "My uncle has a friend whose girlfriend's daughter worked in a doctor's office. She said it's probably a spider bite.")

In most cases the "spider bite" is actually not caused by the bite of a spider. The "bite" of this elusive "spider" is more likely a superficial skin infection, abscess, or boil due to one (or more) of the following:

- Splinter
- IV drug needle
- Mosquito bite
- Bee sting
- Ingrown hair
- Shaving accident
- Bite wound (human, cat, dog, squirrel, antelope…)
- IV drug needle
- Poison ivy
- Bug bite (possibly a spider, tick, chigger, flea, scabie, etc.)
- Anything else that breaks the skin and allows bacteria in.

Clinical Indicator:

Term:
Suitcase Sign

Definition:
This clinical indicator is most helpful to emergency medical services (EMS) personnel. The "Suitcase Sign" can often be assessed from a distance of several hundred feet, typically without even stepping-foot outside of the ambulance or formally meeting the patient. As EMS personnel near the scene of an "emergency" they are sometimes greeted at the curb by a well-appearing patient, suitcase-in-hand. This constitutes a "positive" Suitcase Sign.

The Suitcase Sign is a fast and effective way to evaluate the following:

- Mental status—The patient is awake and alert enough to call 911 and get out to the curb with his/her belongings.
- Judgment and decision-making ability— Patient was able to think ahead and consider what s/he would need for the intended hospital stay.
- Respiratory—Patient was able to walk around his/her house to collect and pack clothing, toiletries, slippers, and family photographs for the hospital stay, then lug these items out to the curb.
- Cardiac—Patient has just packed and pulled eighty pounds of suitcase down the stairs and out to the ambulance... he's already performed his own cardiac stress test.

- <u>Neuro</u>—Packing a suitcase and pulling it out to the curb requires balance, motor strength, and coordination.
- <u>Past medical history</u>—Patient is likely familiar with the medical system and understands what typically happens when s/he goes to the hospital, indicating a long-term physical or mental health problem.

As a caveat, the Suitcase Sign should be interpreted with caution in a sick-appearing patient or in cases where a friend or family-member has packed the bag and assisted the patient to the curb.

Layman's Terms:

One-liners and Such

Thought-provoking statements...

Asthmatic patient complaining of cough and shortness of breath:

"When can I go out and smoke?"

Commentary:
I was going to suggest a neb treatment, but hey, maybe inhaling fire will work better...

(Note: If you were offended by the above statement, please consider reviewing the "Introduction" chapter. If you found the statement funny, keep reading.)

Upon telling a patient she is pregnant:

"I'm pregnant?! How did that happen??!!"

We can explain it in detail if you'd like…

The morbidly obese patient with a blood sugar of 350:

"I'm diabetic. I need to eat!"

Wait, isn't that part of the problem?

(Say the above statement aloud, see if you can find the hidden pun)

"I'm taking too many milligrams! I'm taking a lot more milligrams than my wife."

The patient had added up the total number of milligrams of every different medication that he takes and compared that number to the total number of "milligrams" taken by his wife.

Similar statements have been heard from a few different patients. Remember, it's not the size of the "milligram" that matters...

Patient's chief complaint: "Severe tooth-pain"

Patient's first question: "When do they serve lunch around here?"

*Yikes. This patient wants to eat hospital food **by choice**? The toothache is going to be the least of his problems...*

So close…

Paramedics' call to medical control:
"We have an unconscious male on the front steps of a bakery with a blood sugar of 23"

…yet, so far

A woman in the community, discussing her thoughts of a breast cancer research foundation:

"I'm a [cancer] survivor but I'm not gonna donate any money to the foundation. They already have millions of dollars and they haven't found the cure yet."

I'm not even sure how to comment on this one. The best comment would probably include a statement of disbelief mixed with a side of sympathy.

Triage nurse: "Your family can come back with you, but your girlfriend will have to wait in the waiting room."

'Girlfriend': [Kisses patient]

Patient: "But she's my sister."

Ok, I'll admit it, this one isn't all that funny. However, I have a special connection to this quote…I was the patient. I figured that the appearance of an incestuous relationship was better than forcing my girlfriend (and future wife/physician) to sit in the waiting room. Please try to keep your patients comfortable, even if that means bending the nonsensical rules a little.

Emergency department waits and overcrowding are a major problem. A patient, frustrated with the waiting time, really put things into perspective with this profound statement…

"This wait is ridiculous! If someone was gonna die they'd be dead already!"

Some alternate names I've heard for a gynecologic exam room:

- Pelvitorium
- Bush Gardens

May I also suggest:

- Specularium

A new mother explaining the risks of using a microwave oven:

"I hate microwaves. They cause cancer. I have one, but I only use it to heat up my baby's formula."

Perceived cancer risk versus warm milk: Hmm, tough choice...

"Gangrene runs in my family."

I've never heard of familial gangrene, but then again, I'm no geneticist.
Perhaps generations of uncontrolled diabetes are playing some sort of role here…?

The hypertensive, morbidly obese, hyperglycemic, diabetic patient complaining of chronic knee and back pain:

"Is it ok if I walk over to McDonald's while you wait for my test results?"

And the vicious cycle continues...

Tests *not* to order:

- Stool velocity

- Flatus concentration levels

- Merkin density *(Look it up. Odd, huh?)*

- PR challenge

- Sneeze dispersal rate

"But I need the percs for my L7 disk herniation!"

This patient is either really tall, or has a tail...

(Anatomy Review: There are usually only 5 lumbar vertebrae)

"When I'm in the hospital I always order extra food. The food is really good, and Medicaid pays for it. Well, I don't know. Someone pays for it, but its not me…[giggling]."

The key to fixing our broken healthcare system: Limited access to green Jell-O.

Worst pickup line ever:

Attractive female hospital worker: "Sir, are you an organ donor?"
Male patient: "No, but I could be…" [smile and wink]

Umm, sir, she wasn't referring to that "organ"…

Weird Treatments:

1.) "Sleep with onions in your socks" to cure a fever.

2.) "Vinegar wraps" to reduce bruising and swelling after an injury.

3.) "Duct tape" for laceration repair, fracture immobilization, wart removal, etc.

4.) "Gargle with a mixture of warm water and bleach" for treatment of a sore throat.

5.) "Olive oil" applied to any injured area to prevent swelling.

6.) "Honey" for the treatment of burns and skin infections.

7.) "Alcohol bath" for fevers and poison ivy.

8.) "Vicks Vapo-rub" to cure toenail fungus.

Disclaimer: The above treatments have actually been attempted by patients. However, I do NOT recommend these for actual clinical use. (Although, I think the "onions in the socks" could have some far-reaching public health benefits… isolation would be no problem with the abounding stench of sweaty-onion-feet.)

"I need a pregnancy test. I took 3 home pregnancy tests and they were all positive."

Do hospitals use pregnancy tests that yield a more negative result?

A patient is discharged after recovering from a drunken-stupor. The patient returns, asking:

"Excuse me, can you tell me where I was found?"

Ponder that Descartes...if that's not philosophical, I don't know what is.

"I'm bleeding like a stuffed pig."

I consulted a taxidermist on this one...interestingly, stuffed pigs don't bleed.

Layman's Terms:

In Seriousness...

Finally, something worthwhile! How boring...

Is anyone actually reading this section? If so, congratulations! You made it all the way through the fun part of the book and have ended up at the dull "public service announcement" section…

I hope you have enjoyed and found some humor in this book so far. At this point I would like to take the opportunity and *try* to give this book some sort of redeeming value. The several hundred medical misinterpretations and malapropisms in this book have served as a bit of an eye-opener for me. While writing this book I have again realized how confusing the medical language can be. Although I vaguely recall the frustration of learning medical terminology while in school, the language of medicine has since become a well-rehearsed daily routine. Yet, even with the daily practice I still manage to mix-up and forget medical words quite often. Considering this, I can completely understand how a patient, without any medical background, could have difficulties interpreting the "doctor talk". These interpretation difficulties likely add stress to the clinical environment—both for the patient or family member and the clinician, each trying to figure out what the other is attempting to say.

To help improve the clinical stress, I have tried to change the way I deal with misinterpreted words. When I starting working clinically I would hear the misinterpretations, giggle in my head a little, and move on. Only occasionally would I provide the correct word. It was a tiny bit of seemingly harmless entertainment. However, as time has passed I've started to take a more active role in correcting the misinterpretations. Because of my own experiences, both clinically and with the writing of this book, I felt the need to look slightly beyond the superficial humor of medical misinterpretation.

The next chapter delves deeper into the topic of medical misinterpretation and humor in medicine. The chapter will introduce some very basic research that was undertaken while writing *Layman's Terms*. The research report is organized much like a journal article to efficiently convey the results of the research survey (and to look all professional, or something...). The survey results were obtained with the ethics of *actual* research in mind. As such, this is the only part of the book that I would consider useful for more than just entertainment.

Layman's Terms:

Original "Research"

Something positive came from this book?

Medical Humor and the Misinterpretation of Medical Terms

The misinterpretation of medical terms seems to occur often, as was suggested by the amount of material in this book. Although seemingly common, the misinterpretation of medical terminology is a rarely studied phenomenon. Medical misinterpretations and malapropisms have been introduced in a few journal articles, primarily for entertainment purposes, however research into this topic is lacking. As an example, a popular family practice journal has published articles listing malapropisms; providing an amusing glimpse of the confused medical term.[1] In a 1992 article, Nelson provided one of the first research-like articles with his retrospective review of humorous medical misinterpretations from a pediatric emergency department.[2] A few 'letters to the editor' published in response to the Nelson article revealed both positive and negative opinions, suggesting mixed feelings to Nelson's use of medical misinterpretations as a humorous topic.[3] However, these few letters provide little information about the opinions of a larger medical audience regarding humor in medical misinterpretation.

As a more general topic, the use of humor in medicine has been more often discussed, reviewed, and studied in the medical literature. The value of humor was highlighted over thirty years ago when Norman Cousins, an author who used humor as a form of self-medication, wrote of his own experiences during the course of an illness.[4,5] Although sometimes criticized, Cousins' writings sparked an increased interest in medical humor.[4] Since that time the nursing and medical community has started to embrace and study the value of humor in medicine. Studies and reviews have credited humor for improving patient communication and comfort, the relief of stress and anxiety, as an outlet for frustration, and as an effective tool in medical and nursing education.[4-6] As a treatment and a coping mechanism, humor has taken its place among the prescriptions and scalpels as a valuable asset to the field of medicine.

While the value of humor in medicine seems clear, opinions on the use of misinterpretations as a source of humor are somewhat hazy. Although medical malapropisms have been listed and medical humor has been studied, there is little data showing the relationship between these two topics. The goal of this brief survey was to gain some insight from healthcare professionals into the topics of medical misinterpretation and humor in medicine.

METHODS:

A brief online survey was created to assess participants' experiences with the misinterpretation and misunderstanding of medical terminology. The survey also evaluated participants' attitudes and opinions toward humor in the medical setting. The survey consisted of eight questions, including two demographic questions. Survey participants were recruited by way of postings on three internet medical forums, a social networking site, the book's website, and emails sent to various healthcare professionals. While the emails and social network posting were directed toward specific individuals, the internet forum postings and website were able to reach a more generalized medical audience. The author was blinded to the specific identity of survey respondents.

RESULTS:
Sixty-six (n=66) participants completed the survey.

Demographics:
The participants represented members of several healthcare professions, including: physicians (11%), physician assistants and nurse practitioners (47%), nurses (8%), EMT/paramedics (8%), healthcare students (21%), and professionals from various allied health fields (8%). One respondent does not currently work in the healthcare industry. One physician and one nurse also self-identified him/herself as an EMT/paramedic, both self-identifiers were included in the demographic analysis.

Fifty-seven participants (86%) have worked in healthcare for at least three years, 54% have worked in healthcare for 6 or more years, and 27% of participants have worked in healthcare for 11 years or more.

Prevalence of misinterpretation in medicine:
All survey participants (100%, n=66) have witnessed the misinterpretation or confusion of a medical term at some time. A vast majority (96%) of the participants witness the misinterpretation or confusion of terms at least a few times every week. Forty-one percent observe the misinterpretation of medical terms by patients or their families "a few times everyday".

Correction of misinterpreted word:
Forty-one percent of survey participants attempt to provide the patient or family member with the correct

medical word or phrase 80-100% of the time. A majority of the participants (58%) provide the correct word less than 70% of the time and 31% percent of participants attempt to provide the correct word less than 30% of the time. Seventeen percent of participants typically never attempt to provide correction of the misinterpreted word or phrase.

Effect on patient care:
Eighty percent of participants feel that the misinterpretation of medical terms has an adverse effect on patient care. A majority of participants (56%) have experienced minor problems (such as wasted time attempting to decipher a medication or medical history) related to the confusion or misinterpretation of medical words. Twenty-four percent of participants have seen a "potentially dangerous situation" caused by medical misinterpretation (such as the confusion of a medication or allergy, "Lasix" being confused with "latex" for example).

Humor in Misinterpretation:
A majority of participants (79%) find humor in the misinterpretation of medical words. Seventeen percent consider their feelings "neutral" regarding humor in misinterpretation. Five percent of survey participants do not find humor in the misinterpretation of medical words.

Humor in Medicine:
Nearly all participants (98%) feel that "humor plays an important role in medicine" (62% "strongly agree" and 36% "agree" with this statement). Two-percent of survey participants feel "neutral" about the role of humor in medicine.

<u>Opinions regarding the concept of this book:</u>
Ninety-four percent of participants support the idea of the book (44% "love" and 50% "like" the idea). Six percent of participants "don't care and have something better to do." None of the participants felt that the concept of this book was offensive.

DISCUSSION:
This survey provided some interesting insight into the medical professional's view of misinterpretation in medicine. As was hypothesized, the misinterpretation or confusion of medical words is a very common occurrence. The fact that almost all of the survey participants observe the confusion of medical words a few times each week, and nearly half observe the confusion daily, suggests how common an occurrence it really is. Aside from being common, the clinical ramifications of medical misinterpretation were of special significance. A large majority of participants have experienced clinical problems related to the misinterpretation of medical words, and nearly a quarter of the participants have observed a "potentially dangerous situation" related to medical misinterpretation. Interestingly, although such a large majority have observed misinterpretation-associated clinical problems, nearly a third of the participants rarely provide the correct medical word to the confused patient or family member.

This survey suggested that a vast majority of medical professionals support the use of humor in medicine and a significant majority find humor in the misinterpretation or confusion of medical words.

There were some limitations to this survey that should be addressed. Although professionals from various different medical fields were polled, a relatively high number of PA/NPs and students responded to this survey and a relatively low number of pre-hospital providers and nurses responded. The PA/NP category was not broken down because in many facilities PAs and NPs work in the same or very similar positions. Unfortunately, this survey was unable differentiate between the opinions of physician assistants and nurse practitioners. This survey provides some good information on the opinions of various medical professionals. However, since the overall number of survey participants was relatively low, the ability to fully generalize these findings is somewhat uncertain.

CONCLUSIONS:
Healthcare professionals often observe the confusion and misinterpretation of medical words. Because of the potential problems that can arise from the confusion of medical terms, it is important that healthcare professionals ensure their patients and family members (and other healthcare workers) understand the correct pronunciation and meaning of the medical term.

REFERENCES:
1. Bennett HJ. Children's Medical Malapropisms. *J Fam Pract* 2002;51(11):982.
2. Nelson DS. Humor in the Pediatric Emergency Department: A 20-Year Retrospective. *Pediatrics* 1992;89:1089-1090.
3. Letters to the Editor. *Pediatrics* 1993;91(3):680.

4. Bennett HJ. Humor in Medicine. *Southern Medical Journal* 2003;96(12):1257-1261.
5. Wender RC. Humor in Medicine. *Primary Care: Clinics in Office Practice* 1996;23(1):141-154.
6. Chiang-Hanisko L, Adamle K, Chiang LC. Cultural Differences in Therapeutic Humor in Nursing Education. *Journal of Nursing Research* 2009;17(1):52-61.

Layman's Terms:

Resources

We're at the end…but wait, there's more!

Resources:

Thank you for choosing to read through *Layman's Terms*. I hope you have enjoyed and have found a bit of humor in this book. Please recommend *Layman's Terms* to your friends and coworkers. Maybe this book will even pay off my student loans...or at least help me afford a cup of coffee. Thanks again for your support.

Please check out the bonus information:

Want more Terms? Check out the *Layman's Terms* website:
(www.funnymed.com)

Some other websites I like:

I nearly failed 3rd grade spelling. I wish Dictionary.com existed back then...
(www.dictionary.com)

My favorite non-subscription resources for medical info:
* Pubmed (www.pubmed.gov)
* eMedicine (www.emedicine.com)
* Google and Google Images (www.google.com)

Although I'm a little partial to this book, I'll admit that there's some other funny medical stuff out there. Try Googling "medical malapropisms" or "medical humor". You won't be disappointed. Happy misinterpretings!